*This book is dedicated to all
those who wish to gain strength,
insight, practice in getting to know themselves and in
expressing themselves
a little freer in the world in which they live.*

Living mindfully
day by day

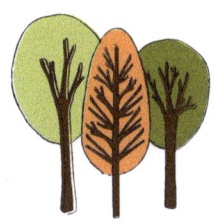

Living Mindfully day by day

"Mindfulness helps you to go home to the present. And every time you go there and recognise a condition of happiness that you have, happiness comes."

— Thich Nhat Hanh

Living Mindfully

Mindfulness is a state you enter when your mind is fully engaged in whatever it is doing in the present moment. You're not thinking about the past or the future - you are totally engrossed in what's happening right now.

You can be mindful at any time of day. If you are new to the practice, try it for five minutes at least once a day. It has a cumulative effect, so don't expect results right away. Make it a habit and you are likely to start feeling more relaxed and in control of your emotions.

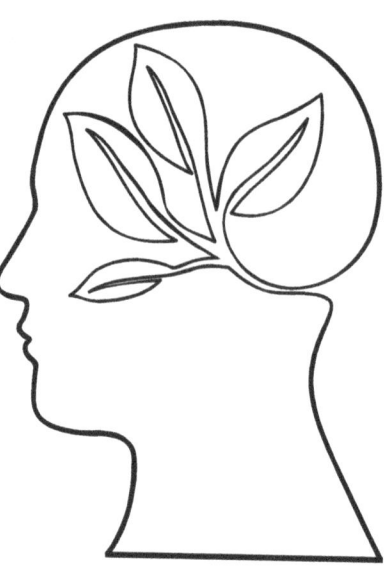

Living Mindfully

REASONS TO BE MINDFUL

- Mindfulness is about living in the moment - being aware of your sensations, thoughts and feelings and the world around you.

- When practised during exercise, it makes the workout more effective because you can focus on the moment rather than be carried away by thoughts.

- You can make it part of your daily routine.

- It can improve your relationships with others by helping you to understand yourself and the trigger that can lead to disagreements.

- You'll feel more confident and your energy levels are likely to increase.

- It will be easier to love yourself.

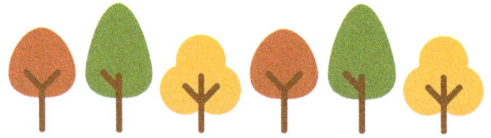

GET INTO A MINDFUL HABIT

Life can often feel fast-paced and full on and it's hard to find time for ourselves when there's so much going on. But we all deserve a few peaceful moments to listen to our own voice and to be mindful.

It's easier to find time than you might think. How many hours do you spend streaming TV shows and movies? How much of your precious time does social media fritter away or time procrastinating over actions or simple things? Can you get up an hour earlier?

There is probably space in your diary for some mindful time and you only need to step away from your busyness for five minutes to notice an improvement in your overall wellbeing.

How to use this book

Begin by spending a few moments reflecting on how you are feeling, both physically and mentally. Consider how both your mind and body feel at this moment in time.

As you read through this book, you'll see that mindfulness is easily practised by turning everyday activities into opportunities for being mindful, to be happier and to appreciate each day.

Within this book are monthly double page layouts providing space to record intentions for the month ahead, self-affirmations to read and recite and other focuses including jottings for sleep and thoughts and feelings.

Enjoy finding your pathway to more energy, joy, fulfilment, freedom and better living.

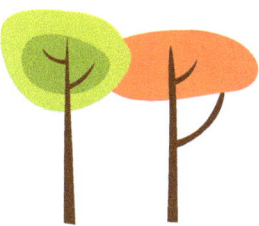

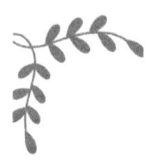 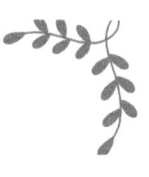

How are you?

Take some time to jot down whatever is on your mind or heart. Think about how you are feeling or what you are experiencing right now in this present moment.

Are you excited about upcoming plans, anxious about a deadline or simply content? Does your body feel rested, achy or energised?

_____
_____
_____
_____
_____
_____
_____

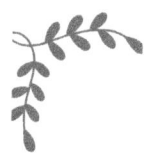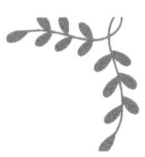

How are you?

_____

_____

_____

_____

_____

_____

_____

_____

_____

_____

LIVING MINDFULLY

in COLOURING

Colouring is a simple and relaxing way of taking time for yourself. It can be a helpful practice if you find it hard to switch off as it allows the mind to slow down and become absorbed without strain.

Try it for yourself with the patterns on the following pages. Take your time selecting the colours you want to use. Then spend a minute or two looking at the intricacies in the patterns before you start. When you're ready, begin to colour.

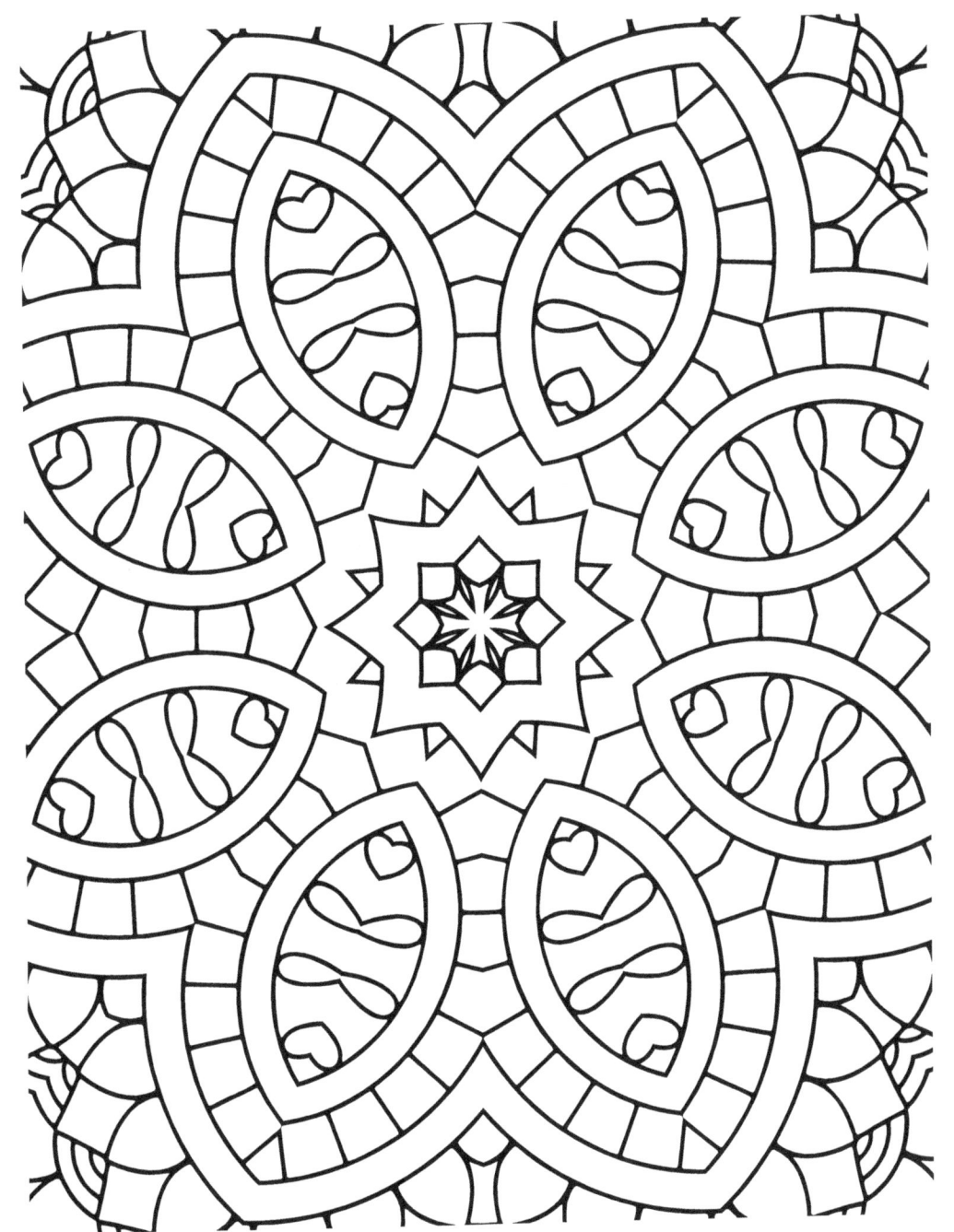

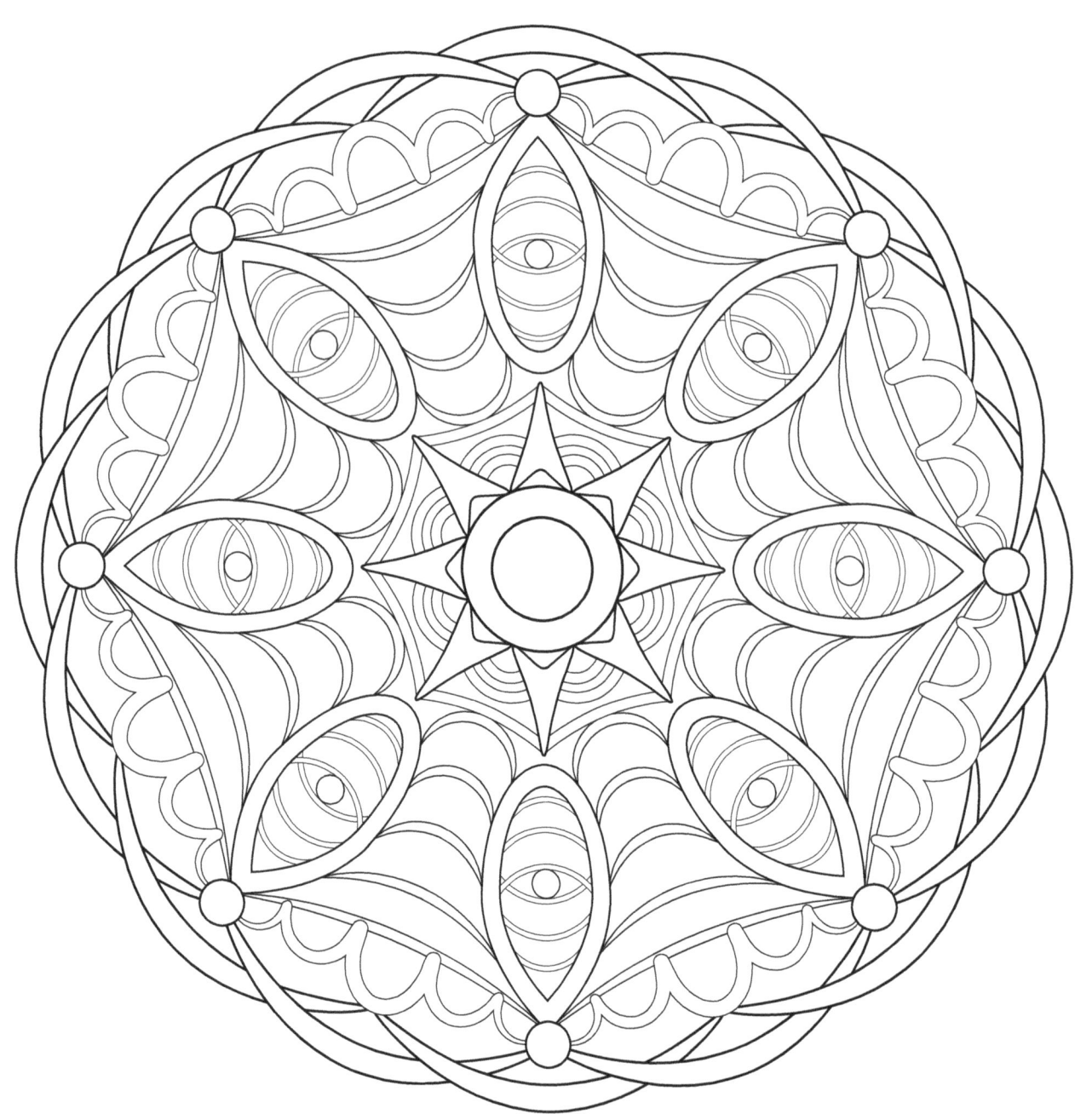

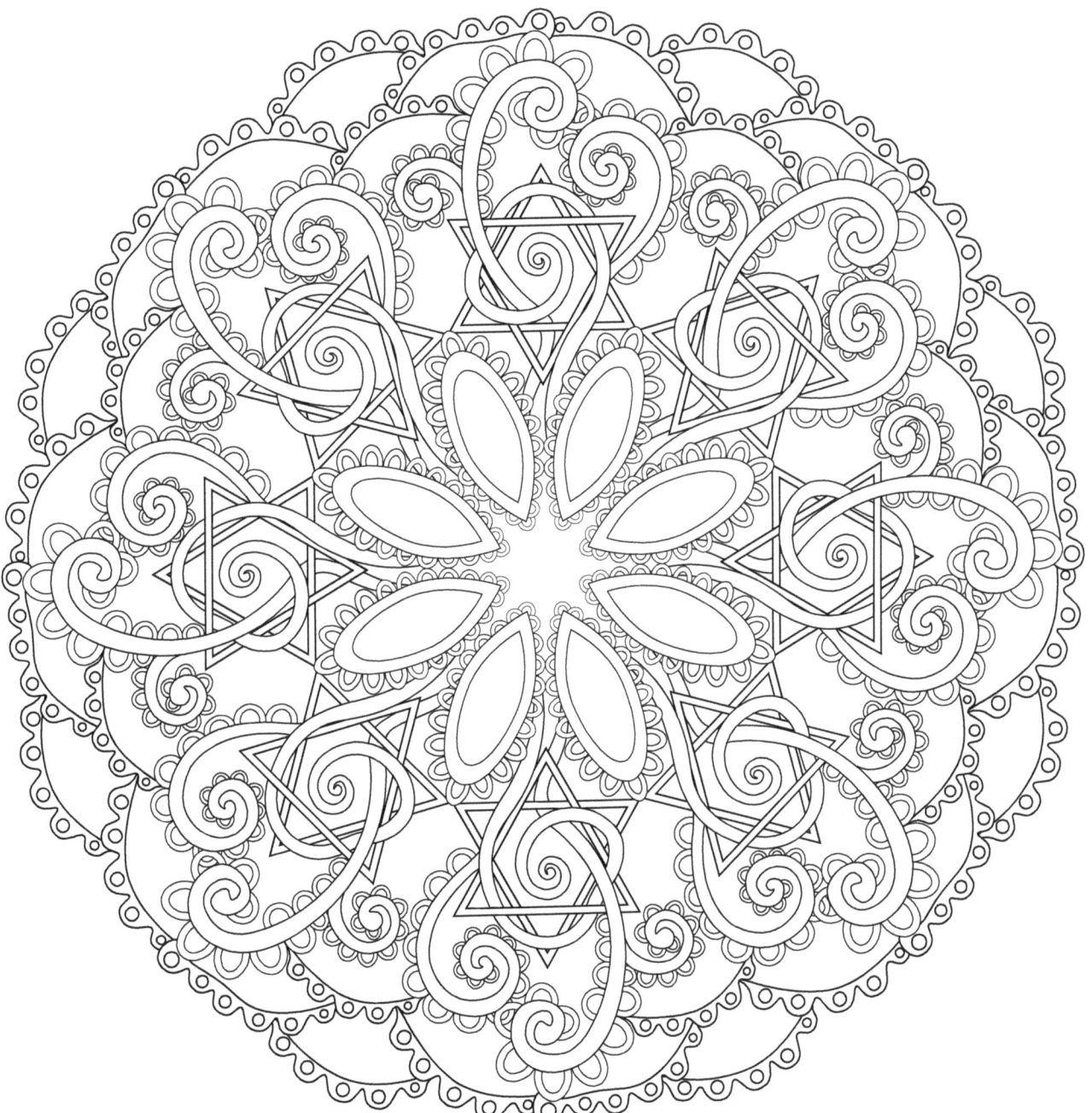

Date _____   J F M A M J J A S O N D

this month's affirmation
ONE DAY AT A TIME, ONE STEP AT A TIME.

Intentions for the month

_____
_____
_____
_____

To do's   Sleep

_____   ☾ _____
_____   ☾
_____   ☾ _____
_____   ☾
                                   ☾ _____
                                   ☾
                                   ☾ _____

Thoughts & Feels

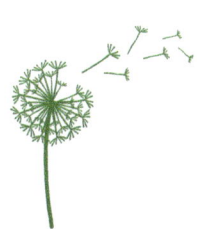

what do you enjoy?

Life can be hectic and many of us don't feel we have time to fit in the things we enjoy. We focus our energy on what we have to do and not what we want to do. And when we have little time for ourselves, we don't tend to give it the attention or respect it deserves.

What do you enjoy doing? Perhaps it's seeing friends, cooking a meal or sitting down with a book. It might be getting into the outdoors on a walk or something more adventurous.

Take some time now to really consider what makes you feel good and write a list here. Then plan for when you're next going to do it.

Doing something new

Creative flow is so important and doesn't have to be too planned or over-thought.

Think about when you last did something for the first time, or something that you used to enjoy, perhaps when you were younger or had more time to endure.

Good things can happen when you make the effort to do something new or when you revisit a hobby or form of enjoyment that can channel your creative flow.

Life can often be hectic and expeditious, where every waking hour is consumed by obligations, deadlines, errands and chores. We often forget to take some time to listen to our own thoughts and feels.

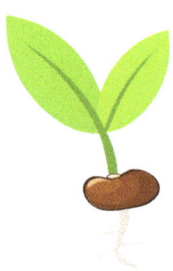

Here are some possible ideas:

- Playing a musical instrument may open up some good vibes and allow you to escape from a moment of displeasure. Being skilled at playing an instrument is a creative outlet that takes time and practice, but whether a novice or not, the pleasure of the moment allows you to switch off mentally and enjoy what your muscles and mind have retained through repetition.

- Visit a place you've never been to. Walk around a part of your town or wander through fields or footpaths you have never explored.

- Try a new food or prepare a new dish for lunch or dinner.

- Learn a new language - possibly from a country you are keen to visit where you can test out your new skills.

- Enrol on a course on a hobby or topic you have always been interested in.

- Try a new activity - a dance class, tennis, a team sport, canoeing, paddle boarding or outdoor swimming.

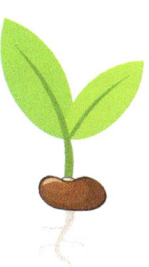

TIPS

What we enjoy doing can change over time so it's worth giving yourself the space to really think about what has recently brought you pleasure.

It can be helpful to think about why you enjoy these things. Is it because they're restorative, creative, energetic? What else could you try that might bring you similar benefits?

"Be happy in the moment.
That is enough."

- Mother Teresa

Date _____   J F M A M J J A S O N D

this month's affirmation
I WELCOME ALL NEW OPPORTUNITIES AND EXPERIENCES.

Intentions for the month

_____
_____
_____
_____

To do's   Sleep

_____   _____
_____   _____
_____   _____
_____   _____
_____   _____
                                _____
                                _____

Thoughts & Feels

_____

_____

_____

_____

_____

_____

_____

_____

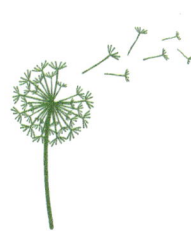

Organise Your Time

Making some adjustments to the way you use your time can be a simple way of helping you to feel more in control of any upcoming plans, events or tasks you're facing and more able to handle pressure.

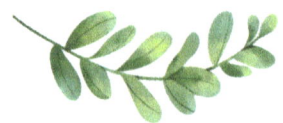

Identify your best time of day - you might be a morning person or an evening person - you do the important things that need the most energy and concentration at that time.

Make a list of all the things you have to do. Arrange them in order of importance and try to focus on the most urgent first. If your tasks are work related, ask a colleague to help prioritise. You may be able to push back some tasks until you're feeling more able to do them.

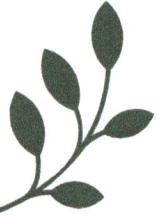

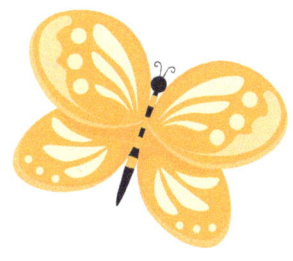

Vary what you do. Balance interesting things to do with more mundane ones and difficult tasks with those you find easier or can do more calmly.

Try not to do too much at once. This seems obvious but we all do it. Multitasking may seem the logical solution but it can sometimes make it difficult to carry out any individual task well. It can also increase the sense of pressure.

Take breaks and avoid rushing. It might be difficult to do this when your're under pressure and feel stressed but it can be more productive. Try to get into the habit of following some of these suggestions and you will feel the benefits of how organising your time can play in your daily life.

LIVING MINDFULLY

in BREATHING

Learning to breathe more deeply can be an easy way of boosting your wellbeing. This is a really simple exercise and works well for when you're in the midst of a difficult day and need a moment to collect yourself.

Breathe in through your nose and out through your mouth. Try to keep your shoulders down and relaxed and place your hand on your stomach - it should rise as you breathe in and fall as you breathe out.

Count as you breathe - start by counting to four as you breathe in, four as you breathe out, then work out what's comfortable for you.

The mind and the breath are profoundly connected. You'll notice that your breathing quickens in times of stress and slows when you are relaxed. Therefore, you will start to feel calmer if you focus on your breathing, slowing it down and taking deeper intakes of air.

When you do this, the heart rate slows, the blood pressure lowers and the body is allowed to rest, which is why breathing properly is an effective stress reliever.

By following a short daily breathing practice into your life, you can expect some of these benefits:

- Reduced stress and anxiety
- The ability to better regulate your emotions
- Improved sleep
- Feeling calmer
- Better posture
- A higher pain threshold

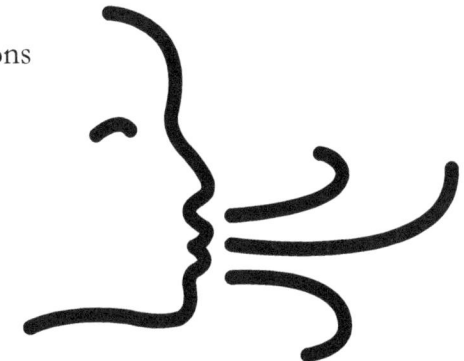

Learning to breathe more deeply can be an easy way of boosting your wellbeing.

If you've got a bit of time, you could move on to colouring the pattern opposite, while keeping your breathing steady.

You could also listen to some calm, soothing music such as sea waves or palm trees gently blowing in the wind.

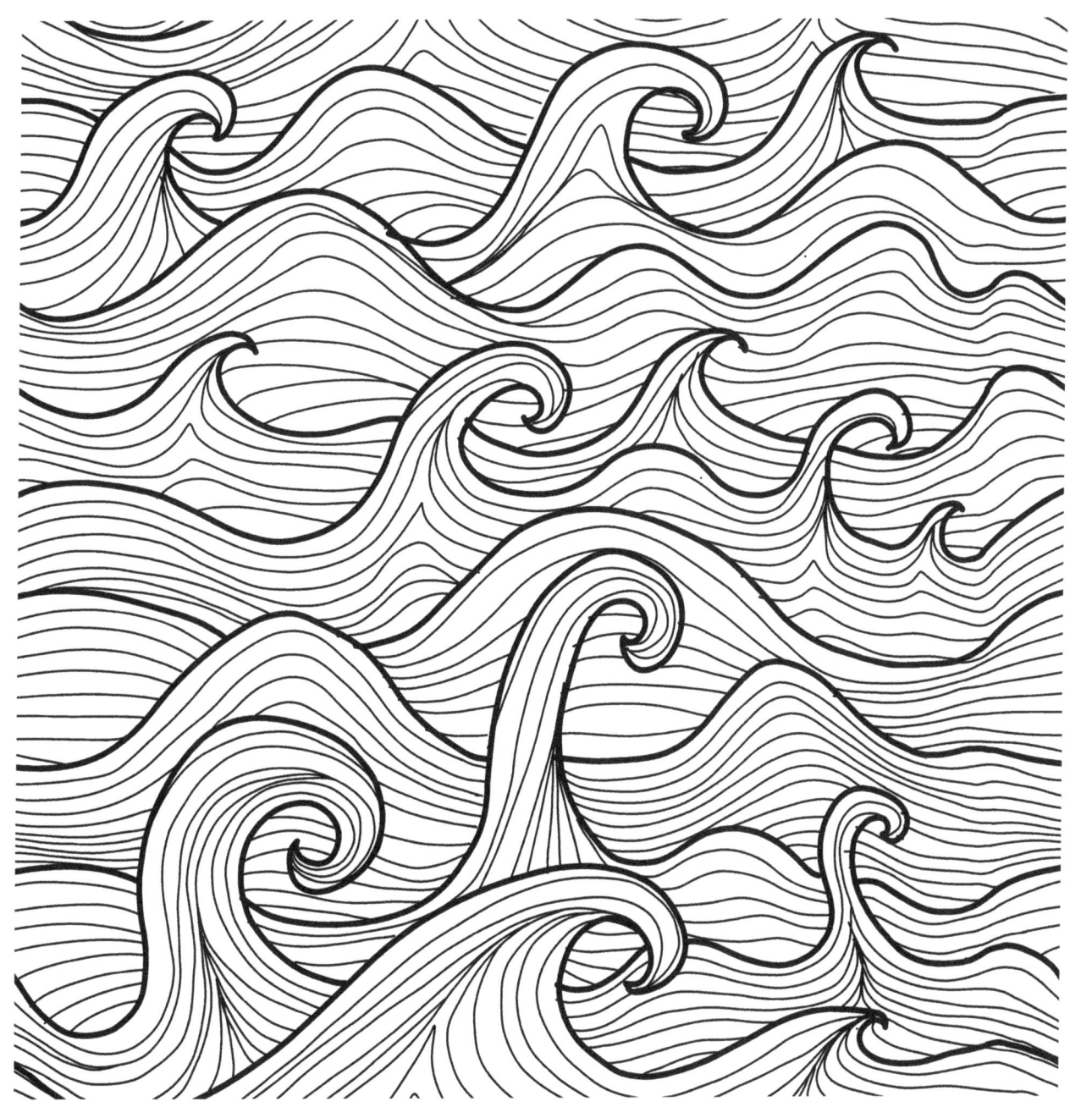

Date _____   J F M A M J J A S O N D

this month's affirmation
WITH EVERY BREATH, I FEEL STRONGER.

Intentions for the month

_____

_____

_____

_____

Sleep

To do's

_____   ☾ _____
_____   ☾ _____
_____   ☾ _____
_____   ☾ _____
                         ☾ _____
                         ☾ _____
                         ☾ _____

Thoughts & Feels

_____

_____

_____

_____

_____

_____

_____

_____

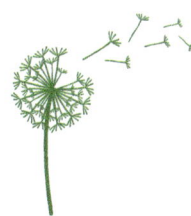

LIVING MINDFULLY

in DAILY RITUALS

Simple moments in life can be injected to bring vast amounts of
joy to your every day - even a simple daily ritual. For example,
taking time to enjoy your morning tea or coffee.

Love this daily ritual from the moment of the preparation to being grateful to enjoying
the flavour and warmth of the first sip while hugging your hands around
the comforting mug or cup.

These tiny moments can become important as you take time
to notice the wonder around you. Experience more of
what life has to offer in daily ritual retreats.

Write down a ritual for yourself on the page opposite.
Take time to love every moment of its magic and pleasure.

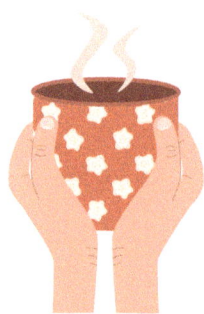

My ritual is:

_____

_____

I enjoy it because:

_____

_____

_____

_____

_____

A mindful activity you can fit into your daily routine is a
tea drinking exercise

If you love drinking tea every day, why not try drinking it a little bit slower? Better yet, try drawing your attention to the sensations, smells or sounds you observe from the moment you start brewing to the moment you finish your cup.

Notice how it feels to make the tea -
- the colour of the tea leaves
- the sound of the kettle
- the wisps of steam from the spout
- the scent that arises
- how it feels in the body as you make and drink the tea.

Tea making and drinking embraces a number of aspects of mindfulness. The process presents a way of being present; focusing, engaging and exercising patience. The ritual can help to slow you down and connect you to yourself.

So when things become rushed, pause and make tea. You could store your tea in an ornate container or perhaps use a special teapot, mug or cup and saucer. Take pleasure in selecting your 'choice' of tea for this moment - soothing peppermint or green tea or something a bit more zesty or zingy like ginger or lemongrass.

Take a sip. Sit calmly and quietly as you drink it. Now and again make a ritual out of tea making.

If you're more of a coffee person, you can perform this practice in the same manner. In fact, you can bring this sort of mindfulness to any activity.

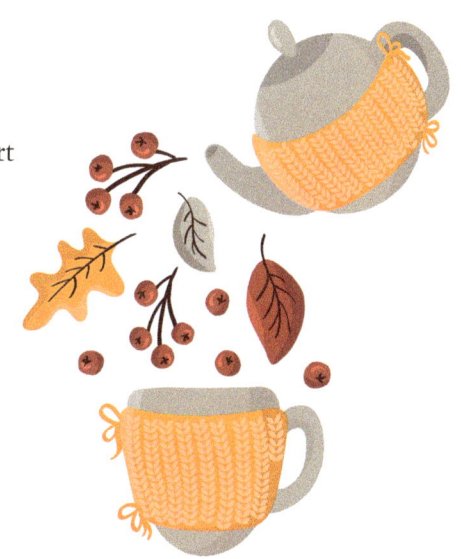

LIVING MINDFULLY

in MEDITATION

Meditation is the practice of calming a busy mind and gently teaching it how to stay centred in among the chaos of everyday life. People who meditate regularly are less stressed, have better concentration and enjoy higher energy levels.

You can meditate anywhere, at any time - all you need is peace and quiet. Ensure that you won't be disturbed as you will be focusing on yourself during the entire experience.

There is no pass or fail with meditating. It will be different every session. Rather than aspire to an outcome, observe what happens with interest.

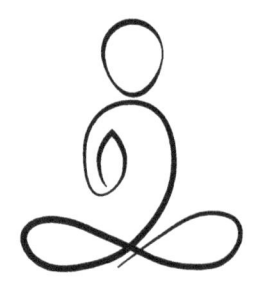

MEDITATION PRACTICE

- Sit comfortably with your back straight and eyes closed.
- Take a deep breath in and exhale slowly. Feel the sensation of the air travelling in and out of your lungs. Do this three times.
- Do a mental scan of your body, starting with your toes and moving up to the top of your head.
- Imagine the tension releasing from each area of your body in turn.
- Count your breaths from one to ten and repeat. If you find it easier, you can repeat one word or a short mantra in your head to focus the mind. An example could be repeating these five words - Release; Peace; Tranquility; Love and Joy.

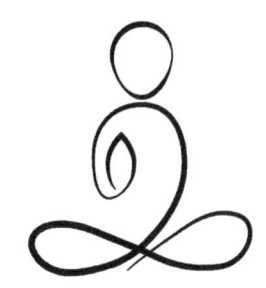

LIVING MINDFULLY
in MINDFUL DRAWING

Take ten minutes to have a mindful experience with drawing. This exercise will provide an act of kindness that will help clear your mind and bring about new perspectives.

Drawing prompts:

1. Focus on your posture. Sit up straight and relax your shoulders.
2. Take a deep breath in for five seconds and then breathe out slowly for five seconds. Repeat this up to ten times.
3. Pick up a pen or pencil and take a moment to focus on your grip. If you find your grip is too tight, loosen it up. Experiment with different ways of holding your drawing tool.

Circles:
- Take your drawing tool and start by slowly drawing a small circle on the page opposite. Don't worry if it's a bit wonky, the point is to pay attention to the process.
- Watch the marks as the pen makes them, feel your hand moving across the page, listen to the sound of each stroke and notice how your body feels.
- Play around with your circles. Vary the sizes between them and create spirals within them. Be sure to fully connect the beginning and end points rather than leaving them unclosed. Take time to focus on what you're drawing. As you notice thoughts arise, let them pass without judgement and bring your attention back to your drawing. Focusing on these sensations can help quieten your mind, like meditation.

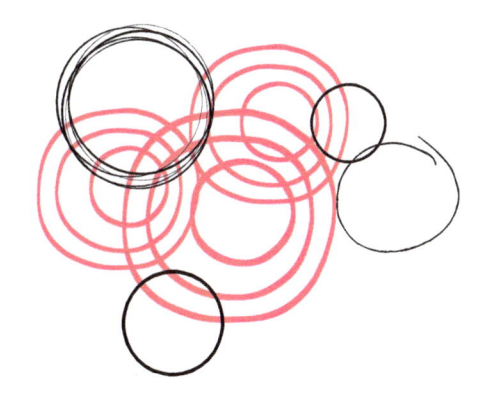

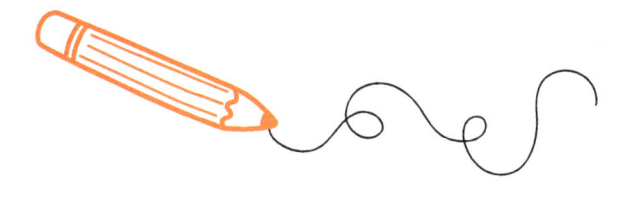

Date _____   J F M A M J J A S O N D

this month's affirmation
I AM LEARNING VALUABLE LESSONS FROM MYSELF EVERYDAY.

Intentions for the month

_____

_____

_____

_____

To do's   Sleep

_____   _____

_____   _____

_____   _____

_____   _____

_____   _____

                              _____

                              _____

Thoughts & Feels

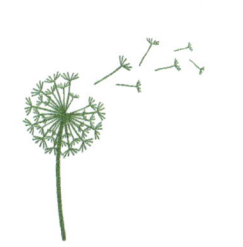

TRY A TEN MINUTE RECHARGE

Just ten minutes away from your hectic life can help you to clear your head and feel calmer and more relaxed.

A good way to start is by simply stepping away, whether it be from the computer screen, your office, chores, dashing around or socialising. You don't have to tell anyone what you are doing - just take a break. Go outside or find somewhere quiet indoors to sit, without your mobile phone to hand.

Take a few deep breaths and imagine you are inhaling energy and exhaling only tightness. Notice what's going on inside. How do you feel? Are there any aches and pains in your body? There's no need to do anything - you're just taking note.

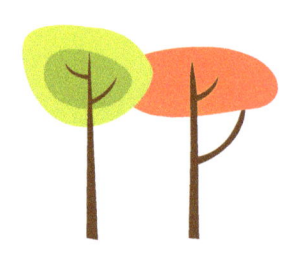

A ten minute walk, preferably outdoors will do wonders for your mood during a busy day - and if you can go somewhere near nature, even better. If you are in the middle of a town, seek out trees or a nearby park.

You can also use your ten minutes as a tea or snack break. Avoid sugary, fatty or overly processed foods for maximum benefits. Likewise, choosing a decaffeinated coffee or tea, or a herbal tea variety is better for you. There's nothing wrong with a good, strong coffee or tea but caffeine is a stimulant and will make it harder for you to wind down.

If there is no way of getting out and you really need a break, find a window with a decent view, open it a little and look out. Allow yourself the luxury of gazing at the scene for ten minutes, noticing all the details out there. If you're wrestling with a problem, sometimes a few moments staring out of the window can encourage the solution to appear.

LIVING MINDFULLY
in GARDENING

Mindful Gardening

Gardening is a great way to practise mindfulness and connect with nature at the same time. Set yourself up with a simple task like planting some seeds, digging some weeds or watering some flowers.

As you do so, place your hand in the soil and feel its texture. Is it rough or fine? Is it damp or dry? Is it warm or cool? Allow yourself to enjoy the process as if you were a child playing.

Notice the weather - not through your mind but through your sensations. Do you have goosebumps from a chill in the air or is there sweat on your brow from the hot sun?

Notice any forms of life around you like a chattering squirrel or chirping bird. You're likely to meet a worm or roly-poly in the soil too.

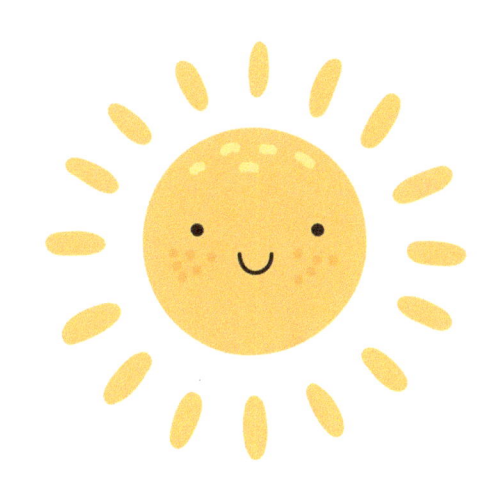

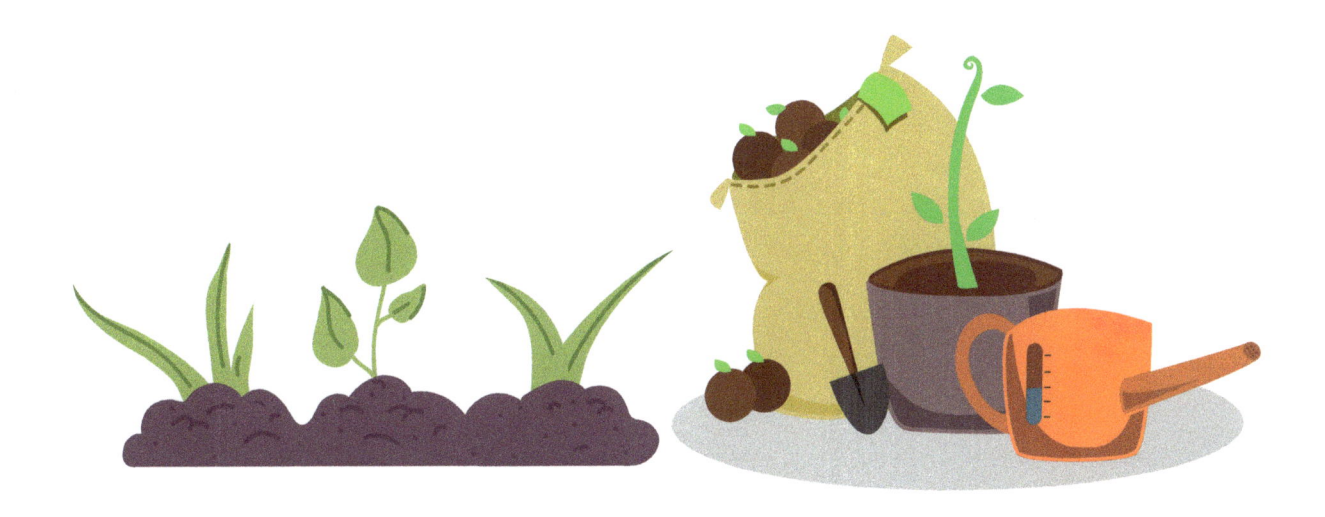

LIVING MINDFULLY
in WRITING

Expressive Writing Exercise

While journaling is all about getting connected with your experiences through writing, expressive writing is about processing emotions. Coping with stressors. Writing exercises let you reflect on meaningful memories and then capture details of the day. It allows you to focus on building confidence as well as reducing troublesome stress ..... without judging yourself for how or what you are feeling.

Expressive writing allows you to channel your stress by writing without stopping. You can later challenge your anxious thoughts, beginning by learning to live in the moment and then take note of the present.

As a guided exercise, recording your thoughts creates space for you to stop after 10 or 15 minutes, look away, take a deep breath and come back to what you've written.

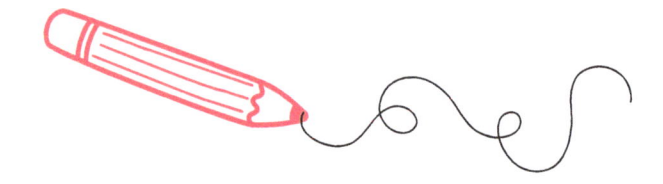

LIVING MINDFULLY
in WRITING

Expressive Writing Exercise

Here's how you can go about accomplishing that feeling, starting with finding the best environment to do the exercise.

In a quiet location, turn on soothing, meditative music and then consider and describe one thing you like to do when you're stressed, upset, anxious, or annoyed. Think about what is bothering you at the moment, allowing yourself the chance to feel without judging.

Relax before writing. Hands should be free, eyes shut and ears focused on the music. Like with guided meditation, inhale deeply, hold your breath, and exhale slowly. In doing so, you'll release tension and stress, increase concentration and relax.

Begin writing freely. Allow yourself to prompt memories as you write, focusing on questions that make you mindful of the present calmness. Sense the soothing after perhaps a grueling day and the changes in your breathing as you record one detail after the next. This exercise is powerful, healthy and paramount in reducing worries and stressors.

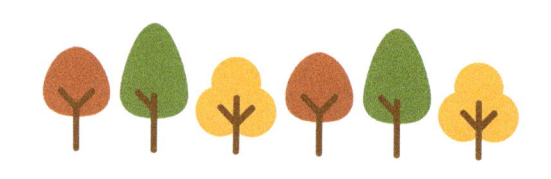

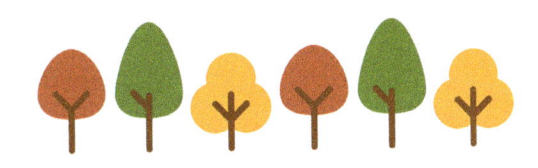

Date _____   J F M A M J J A S O N D

this month's affirmation
I AM LEARNING TO SUPPORT MY BEST SELF.

Intentions for the month

_____

_____

_____

_____

Sleep

To do's

_____   _____

_____   _____

_____   _____

_____   _____

                               _____

                               _____

                               _____

Thoughts & Feels

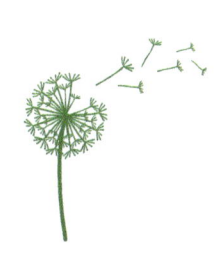

LIVING MINDFULLY

in LISTENING

The goal of any mindfulness practice is simply to experience life as it unfolds. To stay present and calm and not slip back into thinking/worrying mode.

Here we connect to sound so that you can truly experience the moment and a whole lot of other memories with childlike curiosity and without judgement.

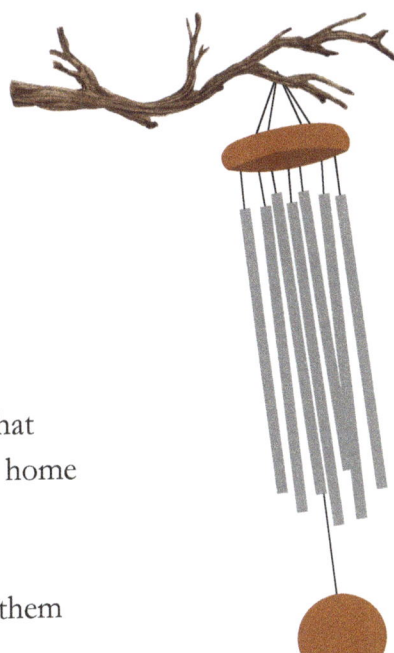

Tune In!

Start with 5 minutes and extend to longer sittings if that feels right for you. Find a spot in a quiet part of your home or garden.

- Take a seat. Now gently close your eyes or keep them in soft-focus (half-closed.)

- Allow sounds to enter your awareness and to let them pass like clouds passing by in the sky, sounds from near and far, coming and going.

- All you need to do is be present to the sound.

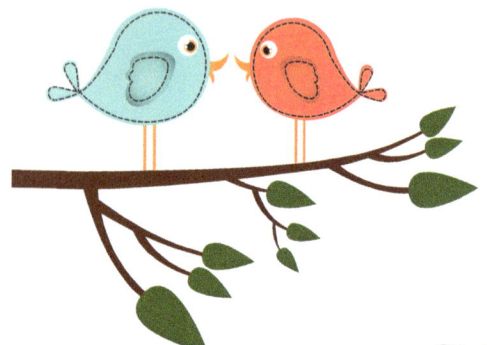

Watching and listening to birds

Birds are all around us; they're a part of our everyday life and our experience of nature. If you take just a little bit of time to look out for and listen to birds - in your garden, in parks, allotments, fields, woods and forests, along riverbanks, at the seaside, in your town and city - you'll soon be aware that there's birdlife everywhere.

The sounds of many species are characteristic and easy to recognise. You'll already know some birds soley by their sounds: the hoot of an owl, the call of a cuckoo. Others - a robin, blackbird, blue tit and sparrow - you will easily recognise by sight.

Start bird-watching just by looking out of your window or sitting somewhere out in the open - the garden, park or street bench.

LIVING MINDFULLY

in LISTENING

Sit patiently for a while. Listen. What can you hear? What can you see? Whether it's up in a tree, high in the sky, on the ground or in a bush, it is more than likely that you will notice a bird or two.

Notice details: their colours, their movements and their behaviour. Watch what they do and where they go. Intrigued? Invite them round to your place; give them food by providing a bird feeder. Be patient. It may take time before you get some visitors.

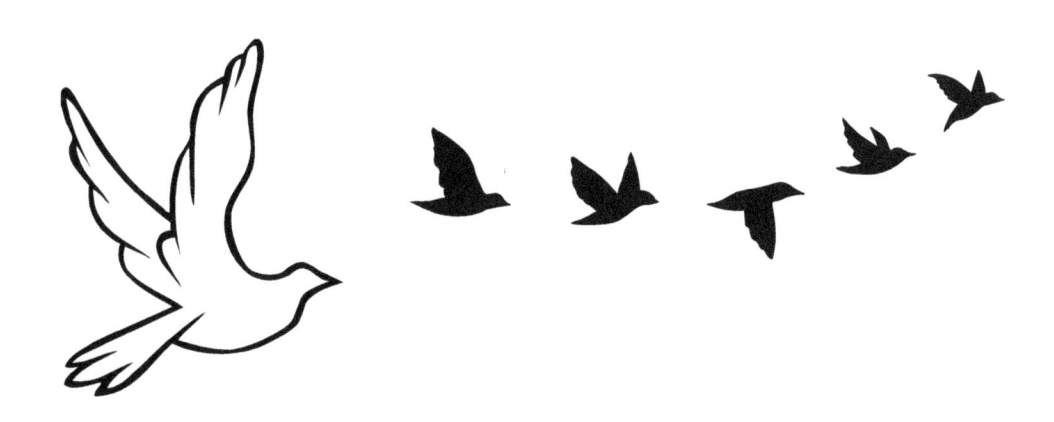

LIVING MINDFULLY

A LITTLE HOW-TO
Colour in the areas of your life that you've focused on lately.

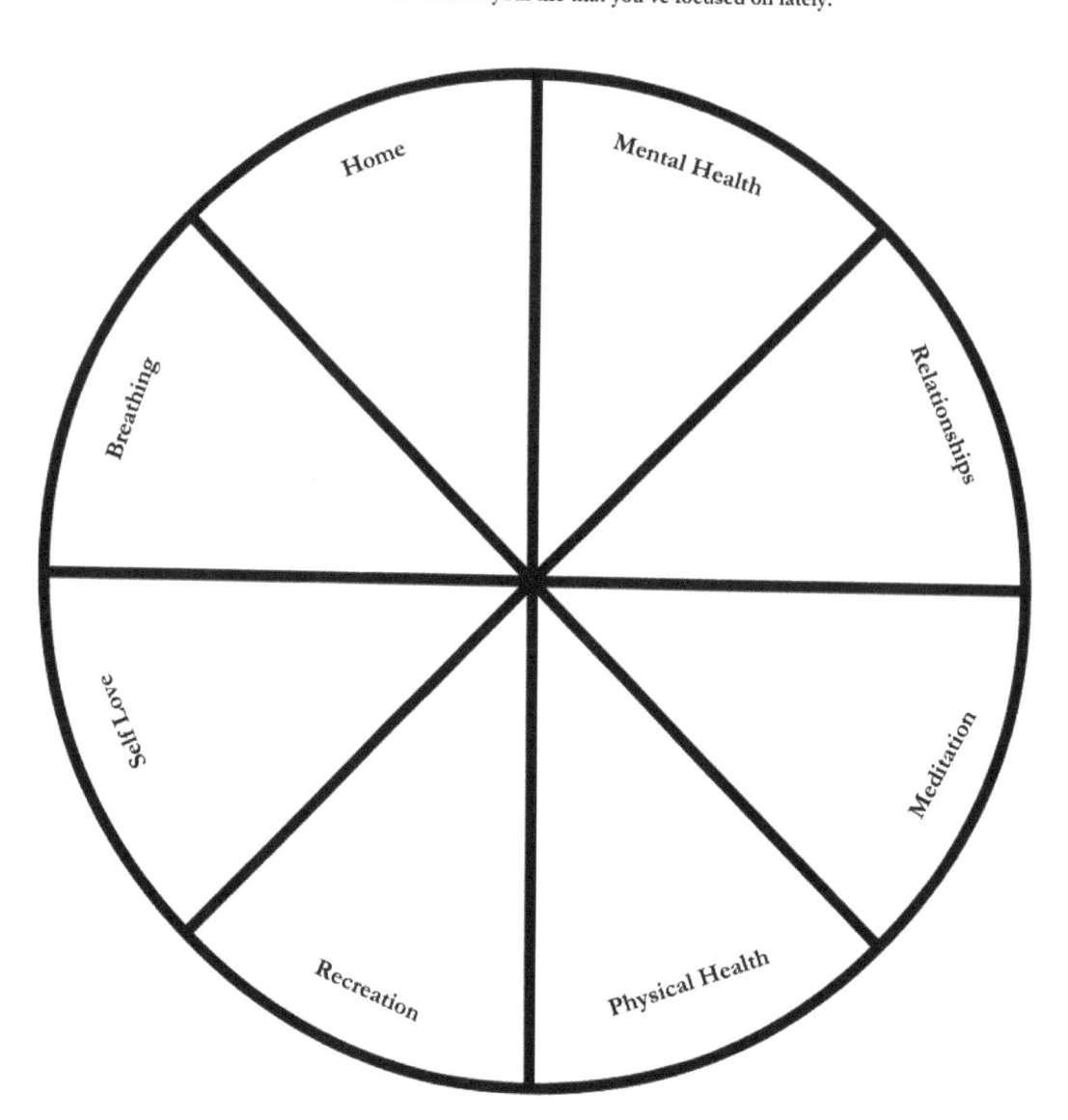

- Home
- Mental Health
- Relationships
- Meditation
- Physical Health
- Recreation
- Self Love
- Breathing

LIVING MINDFULLY

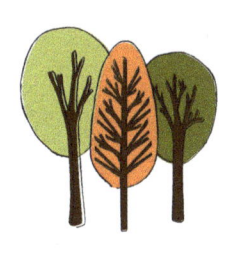

A MINDFUL REFLECTION

Take time to reflect and journal your own mindful moments, experiences and lessons learned.

LIVING MINDFULLY

in POETRY

Mindfulness poetry is a powerful way to connect with the heart of the experience of mindfulness.

Whether or not we have a formal mindfulness practice, mindfulness poetry can help us keep, or regain, our footing in a world of upheaval.

They can inspire you and bring you closer to the wonder of living a mindful and compassionate life.

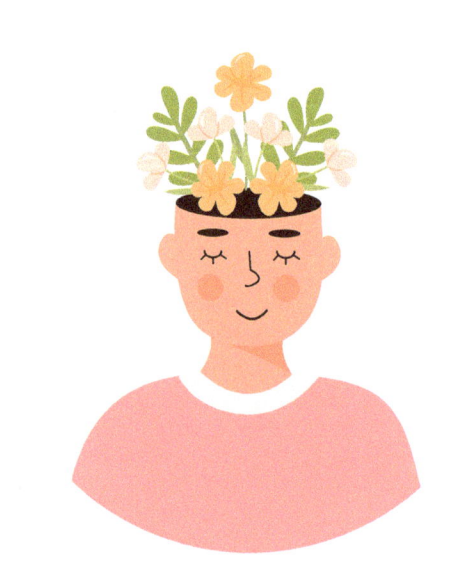

What Do We Know
by Mary Oliver

The sky cleared
I was standing
under a tree.

and there were stars in the sky
that were also themselves
at the moment

at which moment
my right hand
was holding my left hand
which was holding the tree
which was filled with stars
and the soft rain —
imagine! Imagine!
the long and wondrous journeys
still to be ours.

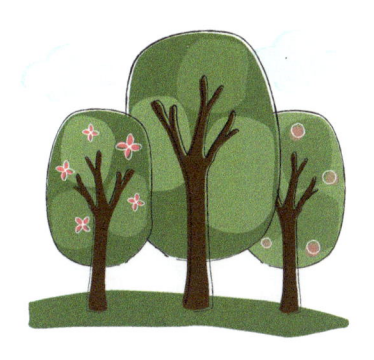

Joy in Life

You must be completely awake in the present
to enjoy the tea.
Only in the awareness of the present,
can your hands feel the pleasant warmth of the cup.
Only in the present, can you savour the aroma,
taste the sweetness, appreciate the delicacy.

If you are ruminating about the past,
or worrying about the future,
you will completely miss the experience
of enjoying the cup of tea.
You will look down at the cup and the tea will be gone

Life is like that.
If you are not fully present,
you will look around and it will be gone.
You will have missed the feel, the aroma,
the delicacy and beauty of life.
It will seem to be speeding past you.

The past is finished.
Learn from it and let it go.

The future is not even here yet.
Plan for it,
but do not waste your time worrying about it.
Worrying is worthless.

When you stop ruminating about
what has already happened,
when you stop worrying about
what might
never happen,
then you will be in the present moment.
Then you will begin to experience joy in life.

Thich Nhat Hanh

Date _____   J F M A M J J A S O N D

this month's affirmation
LIFE DOES NOT HAVE TO BE PERFECT TO BE WONDERFUL.

Intentions for the month

_____

_____

_____

_____

Sleep

To do's

_____   ☾ _____
                                ☾ _____
_____   ☾ _____
                                ☾ _____
_____   ☾ _____
                                ☾ _____
_____   ☾ _____

Thoughts & Feels

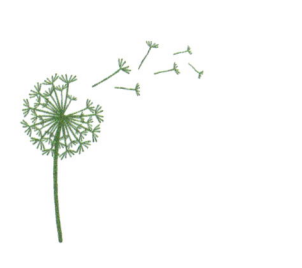

_____

_____

_____

_____

_____

_____

_____

_____

LIVING MINDFULLY

Give Yourself A Break

Learning to be kinder to yourself in general can help you control the amount of pressure you feel in different situations.

Reward yourself for achievements - even small things like finishing a piece of work or making a decision.
You could take a walk, read a book, treat yourself to your favourite food or simply tell yourself 'well done.'

When you're feeling low, look back at the list you wrote for 'What Do You Enjoy?' and make a plan to do at least one of those things in the next few days.

LIVING MINDFULLY

Give Yourself A Break

If you are lucky enough to have access to a garden, it will make the outdoor sanctuary for all kinds of mindful activities - from quiet contemplation through to yoga, gardening, reading or dozing in the sunshine.

A spot of gardening can be extremely therapeutic and a water feature can be a lovely addition to any setting. The tranquil sounds of trickling water can be so soothing as you watch wildlife plunging in pools or splashing in birdbaths .

Spending time in a garden will provide pleasure all round. The smells, sights, sounds and sensations will create a wonderful world of wellbeing. You don't need a huge amount of space - a small balcony is enough to create a zone where all your senses can be stimulated.

THE BEAUTY OF
GRATITUDE

"The quality of being thankful; readiness to show appreciation for and to return kindness."

Can happiness bring gratefulness? Can gratefulness bring happiness?

Much of life is made up of a collection of happenings and fleeting moments - of kindness and appreciation. You feel gratitude when you are aware of and acknowledge those happenings and moments.

At any one time, when you appreciate what is good in life, you will receive a positive feeling of connection with the world around you. During difficult and challenging times, when you may feel sad, upset, worried or anxious, being aware and acknowledging the good things, when and where they occur, can help comfort you.

Starting each day reflecting on those things that we are thankful for and taking stock of what we do have can help us refocus on the positives in our lives and give some helpful perspective. Whether it's gratitude for a warm, close friendship, a beautiful sunny day, hearing birds twittering, a sleeping kitten or simply having that first delicious morning brew, it all counts and we can focus on the good things in life.

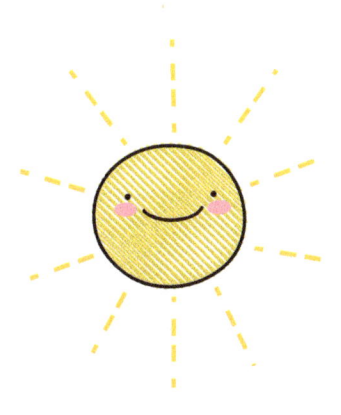

Take a few moments to write down some things you are grateful for in your life.

I am thankful for

....

I am thankful for

....

I am thankful for

....

Get in the habit of noticing and reflecting on the small pleasures of what life brings you. You may simply wish to reflect on what those things are at the end of each day. Make a point of looking for things to appreciate day by day and you will discover this practice will remind you that this positive feeling of connection is hidden in every minute of each day.

"I am happy because I'm grateful. I choose to be grateful. That gratitude allows me to be happy."

— Will Arnett

LIVING MINDFULLY

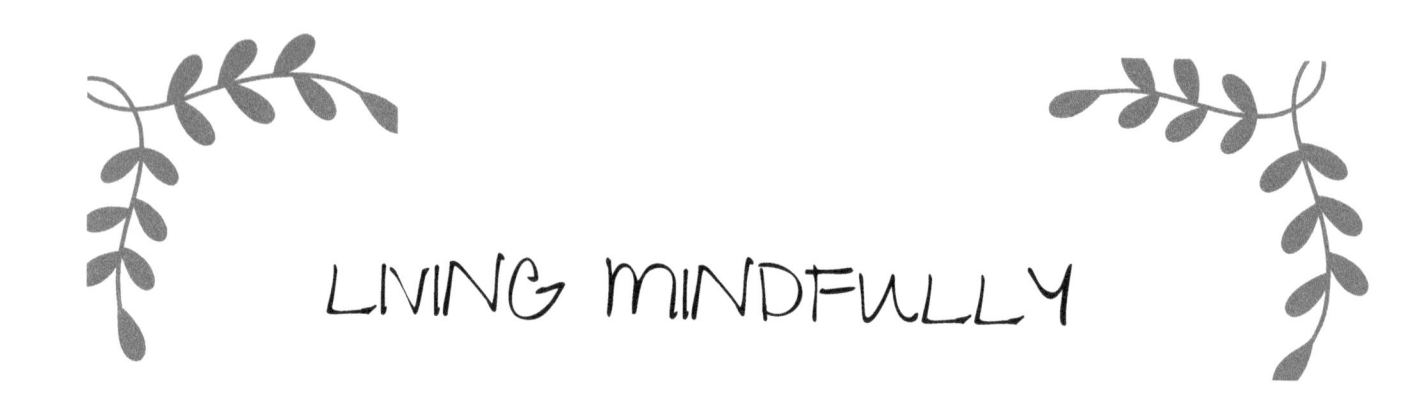

Spending time outside and in green spaces can be great for your physical and mental wellbeing. To get the benefits you could:

Go for a walk in the countryside or through a local park, taking time to notice trees, flowers, plants and animals you see on the way.

If you don't have time to go out into nature now, bring some of the power of green things inside by colouring the page opposite using different shades of green.

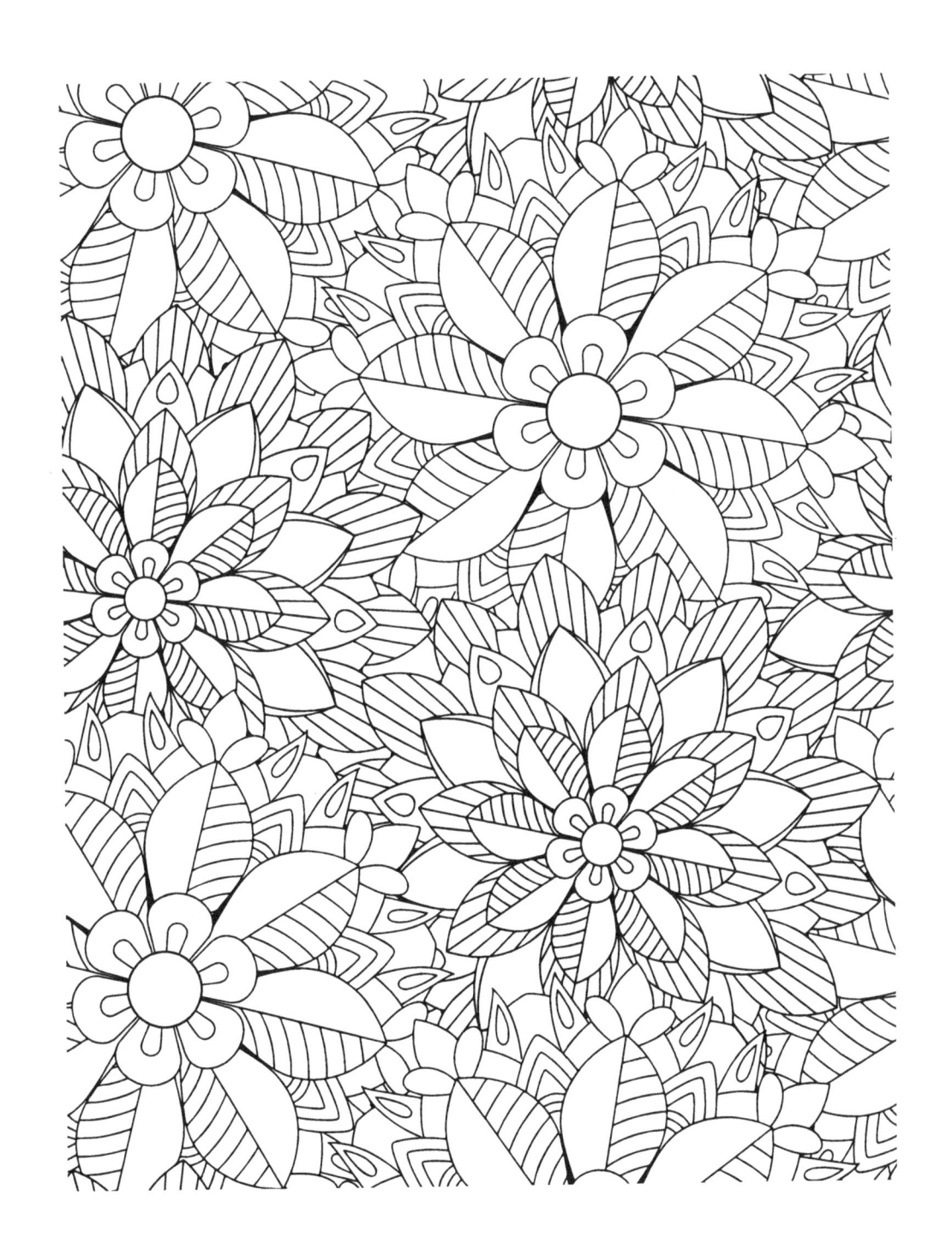

Date _____   J F M A M J J A S O N D

this month's affirmation
I AM EXCITED TO WAKE UP EVERY DAY AND EXPERIENCE THIS BEAUTIFUL LIFE THAT I AM CREATING WITH MY THOUGHTS AND VISIONS.

Intentions for the month

_____
_____
_____
_____

To do's   Sleep

_____   ☾ _____
_____   ☾ _____
_____   ☾ _____
_____   ☾ _____
                               ☾ _____
                               ☾ _____
                               ☾ _____

Thoughts & Feels

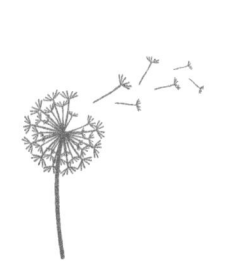

LIVING MINDFULLY

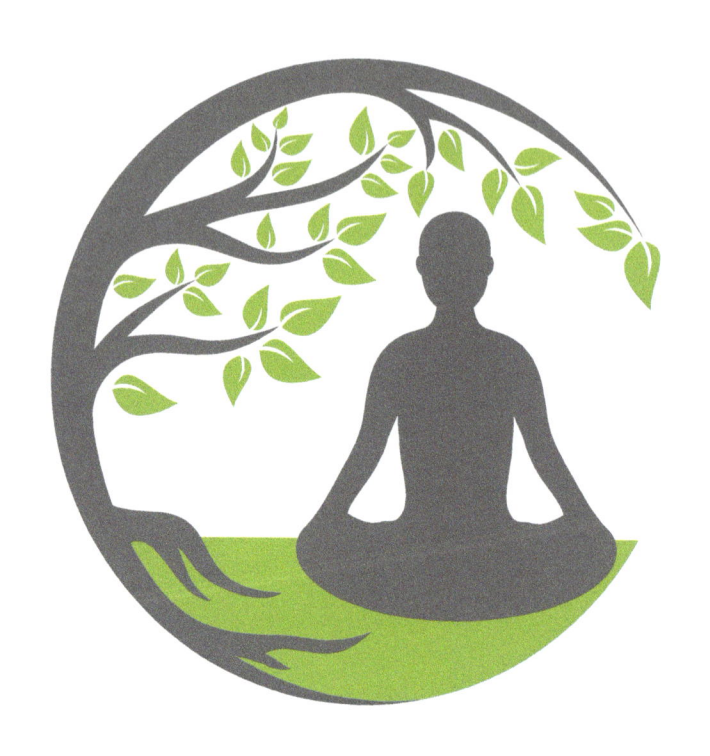

in NATURE MEDITATION

LIVING MINDFULLY

in NATURE MEDITATION

Meditating outdoors, close to nature, can be relaxing,
inspiring and healing. It will give you a boost if you manage
to do it regularly. Green spaces are mood-enhancing.

It's as simple as sitting somewhere quiet,
where you can hear the wind in the trees and the birds singing.
You could find a spot in the countryside, on a beach or even in
your own garden. As long as nature is close by and it is peaceful,
you will feel wonderfully soothed by being outdoors among
trees, plants and animals.

We are part of the natural world. It is all around, in the streets, buildings, towns and
cities. Wherever we are, it is always there.

LIVING MINDFULLY
in NATURE MEDITATION

- Find a place outdoors to sit comfortably.

- Take three deep breaths and become aware of your body. Feel the grass or ground beneath you and do a quick body scan from your toes to the top of your head. If you can, take off your shoes and socks and touch the ground beneath your feet.

- Keep your eyes open and look at the nature around you.

- Feel the sun, breeze, cold or warmth on your face.

- Listen to the sounds of nature - the birds, the rustle of leaves, the creaking of trees.

- Breathe slowly and deeply. Continue to take in your surroundings. If you feel comfortable, you can deepen this meditation by closing your eyes. There is no time limit to this but it's best to do this for at least ten minutes.

LIVING MINDFULLY

in NATURE MEDITATION

"Whenever your mind becomes scattered, use your breath as the means to take hold of your mind again."

— Thich Nhat Hanh

LIVING MINDFULLY
in MINDFUL DRAWING

Take ten minutes to have a mindful experience with drawing. A big part of meditation is focusing on the breath, noticing how long each breath is and what is feels like as you inhale and exhale.

Drawing prompts:
1. Focus on your posture. Sit up straight and relax your shoulders.
2. Take a deep breath in for five seconds and then breathe out slowly for five seconds. Repeat this up to ten times.
3. Pick up a pen or pencil and take a moment to focus on your grip. If you find your grip is too tight, loosen it up. Experiment with different ways of holding your drawing tool.

Draw the Breath

- Take your drawing tool and start on the edge of the page in the middle.
- Gently move your pen up and down the page, syncing it with your breath. As you breathe in, make a mark moving up the page. When you get to the top of the breath, make a small curve before bringing your line down the page as you exhale.
- Make a small curve at the bottom of the breath before moving the pen back up your paper. Don't try to control your breath. Let it flow naturally and simply be aware of it. When your mind wanders, notice it and bring your awareness back to the page.

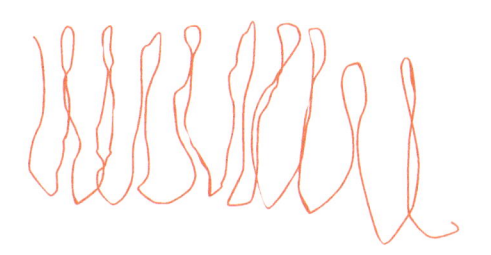

You're likely to notice the lines extending a bit longer as you become more present and calmer. You may also notice different patterns each time you do it, depending on how you're feeling at that moment.

Date _____   J F M A M J J A S O N D

this month's affirmation
I TRUST MYSELF TO MAKE THE RIGHT DECISIONS.

Intentions for the month

_____

_____

_____

_____

To do's   Sleep

_____   _____

_____   _____

_____   _____

_____   _____

                              _____

                              _____

                              _____

Thoughts & Feels

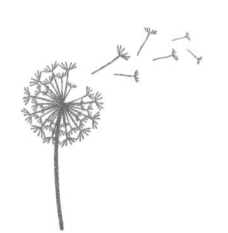

_____

_____

_____

_____

_____

_____

_____

_____

LIVING MINDFULLY

in SELF LOVE

Living Mindfully involves the process of learning to love yourself. Self-love is about more than feeling good; it's about being your own biggest fan.

Get to know yourself. Sit quietly and ask: "How do I feel?" What's going on with your emotions? Relax and invite them in. If negative emotions surface, don't panic - they will pass through and be released, if you don't resist them.

Self-care. Look after yourself. It is possible to put yourself first without being selfish. If you don't meet your own needs, how can you be expected to look after anyone else's?

LIVING MINDFULLY

in SELF LOVE

Set clear boundaries: Don't allow yourself to be coerced into doing things you'd rather not. Be honest with others and don't worry too much about what other people think.

Be kind to yourself: Treat yourself the way you would treat others. Accept you are in charge of your own destiny: Actively choose the kind of life you want to live and follow your dreams. Yes, there will be setbacks and things might not always go your way but with the right mindset, you can achieve anything.

Avoid toxic relationships: You don't need to take on anybody else's problems or put up with toxic behaviour. Treat yourself like a god or goddess who only deserves the best and won't accept anything less. Don't be unkind but be firm and make sure you spend the majority of your time with those who love you and make you feel good about life.

LIVING MINDFULLY

in SELF LOVE

If you have a bit of time, why not reflect on your feelings about self love while colouring the pattern opposite.

Remember, colouring is a simple and relaxing way of taking time for yourself.

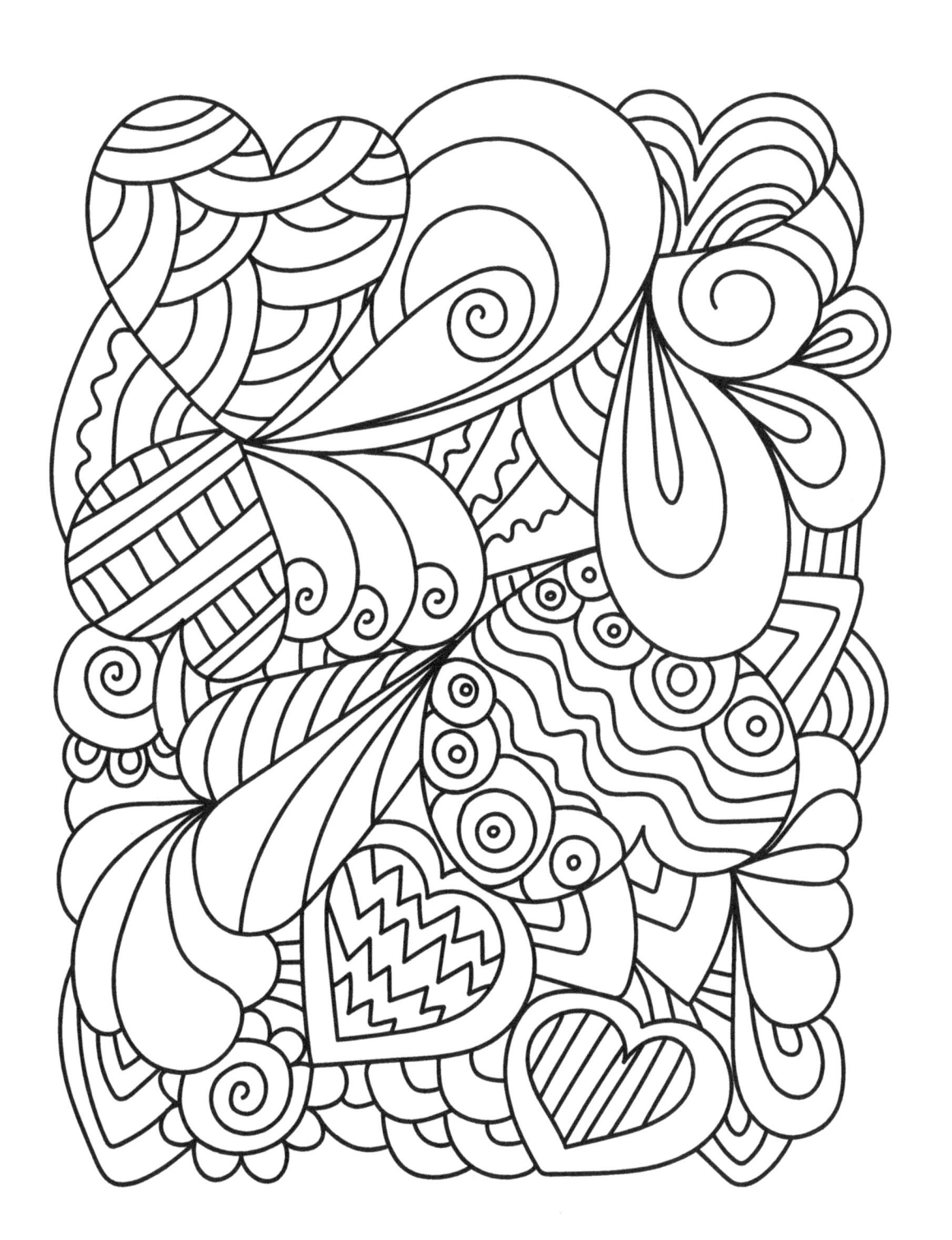

LIVING MINDFULLY
in WALKING MEDITATION

You can also try meditation while walking. This can happen anywhere but it is particularly good when done close to nature. For Buddhist monks, walking is an essential part of their practice and they often do it for as long as 15 hours a day, however, ten to fifteen minutes spent walking in nature is enough for a deep and relaxing experience.

Walking meditations can focus, engage and harmonise your body, breath and mind. Just walk at the speed and pace that keeps you focused and engaged with the physical experience of walking and try not to think about other things.

It takes some practice but once you have mastered it, it clears the mind, reduces stress and can create a feeling of inner calm.

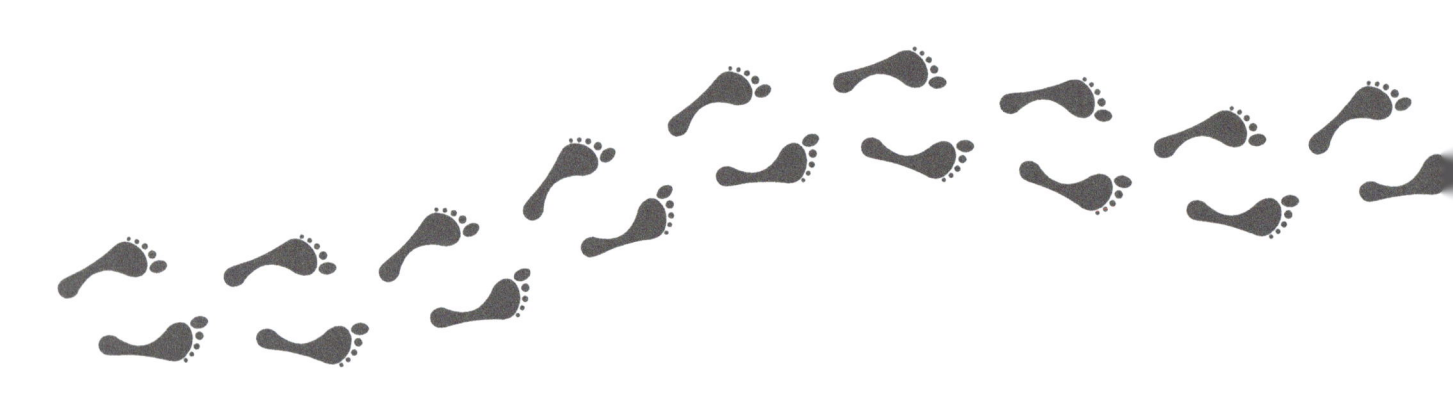

LIVING MINDFULLY

in WALKING MEDITATION

- Choose a secluded, pretty spot you are going to walk back and forth on the same path.

- Take three deep breaths and pay attention to the sensation of your feet on the ground.

- Start to walk slowly, at least half your normal pace. As you move, place all of your attention on the soles of your feet.

- Walk back and forth along the same stretch, not looking at anything in particular.

- If your mind wonders, bring your attention back to the sensations and motion of your feet.

- If at any time you feel like standing still or sitting, then do so.

- If something beautiful catches your eye stop to look at it.

- There is no "correct" experience. Just keep walking and if any difficult emotions surface, allow them to pass through.

- As you walk, enjoy every step you take and feel gratitude for the natural world around you.

Date _____   J F M A M J J A S O N D

this month's affirmation
I LET GO OF OLD, NEGATIVE BELIEFS THAT HAVE STOOD
IN THE WAY OF MY SUCCESS.

Intentions for the month

_____

_____

_____

_____

Sleep

To do's

_____   _____

_____   _____

_____   _____

_____   _____

                                                        _____

                                                        _____

                                                        _____

Thoughts & Feels

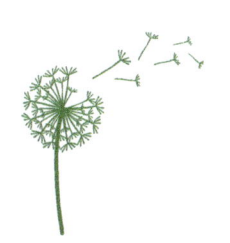

_____

_____

_____

_____

_____

_____

_____

_____

Mindful Eating Every Day

Each meal of the day can be a call to mindfulness and
gratitude. We often eat mindlessly, rushing to eat too quickly
at our desk or lounging in front of the TV. When life is fast,
eating quickly or on the go can become the norm. As a result,
it creates a disconnection between ourselves and the food that nourishes us.

Eating slowly is about the experience of sourcing, preparation and
enjoying the whole process.

Slowing down to cook, eat and drink intentionally are part
of developing a healthier relationship with food.

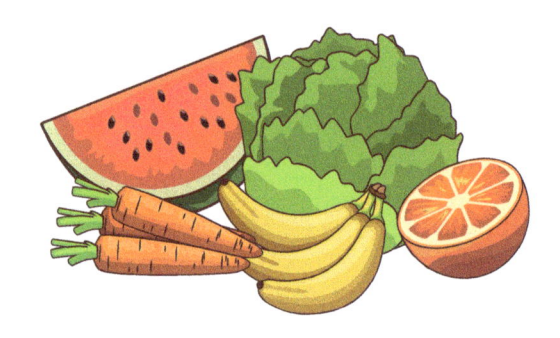

When you have some free time, gather some fresh ingredients together and mix up a salad to serve on the side or as a main course. You may find that preparing meals - grating, chopping, stirring and arranging can have a significant effect in how the processes quietens the brain and brings a peaceful air to the environment in which you are present.

Mindful eating is a way to turn something you do everyday into a mindfulness practice. Take time to enjoy your food and you'll more likely to notice flavours and textures.

It can take your body up to 20 minutes to register the fact that you are full but during that time you may be continuing to eat. Check and ask yourself, "Am I still hungry or am I full?"

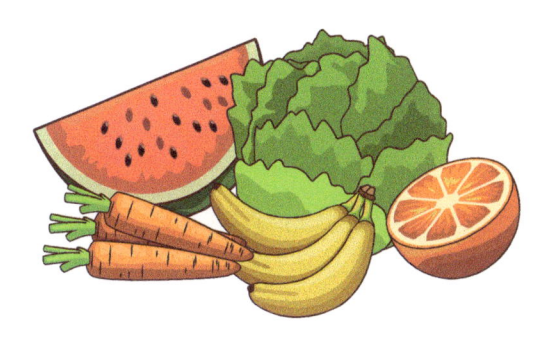

Mindful Eating Every Day
– some Recipe inspiration

Here are two nutritious recipes to try. The Berry Smoothie can be enjoyed as a breakfast for a delicious start to the day or for a healthy pick me up some time later.
The pancakes would make an ideal brunch or afternoon treat!

BERRY SMOOTHIE

This smoothie is full of goodness and can be adapted to use any yogurt or frozen fruit. Vegan yogurt alternative can also be used.

Preparation Time: 10 mins.   Serves 4
- 350g mixed berries
- 2 ripe bananas
- 250g yogurt
- 100g rolled oats
- 4tbsp chia seeds

1: Put all the ingredients into a large blender with 500ml cold water.
2: Whizz until smooth.
3: Divide between 4 glasses and serve.

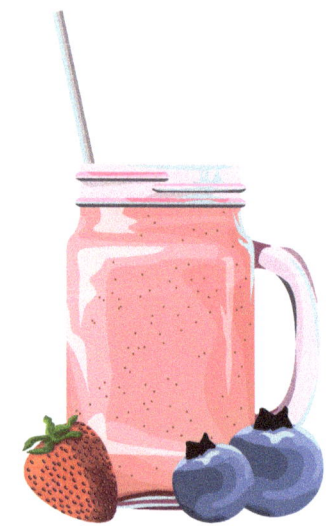

Mindful Eating Every Day
– some Recipe inspiration

BANANA OAT PANCAKES

Easy, flourless and sugar-free, these pancakes are a healthy and satisfying snack, whatever time of day.

Preparation Time: 5 mins. Cooling/Cooking Time: 20-25 mins. Makes 3-4 pancakes

- 1/2 Cup of rolled oats or old fashioned oats. Instant oats and steel cut oats won't work.
- 2 bananas
- 2 eggs
- 1/2 teaspoon baking powder
- Pinch of salt
- Maple syrup to serve (optional)
- Fresh fruit of your choice to serve

1: In a blender, combine the peeled bananas, eggs, oats, baking powder and salt.
2: Blend until the mixture is smooth to form a batter.
3: Allow the batter to stand for 10-20 mins until thickened slightly.
4: Heat a non-stick frying pan over a medium heat.
5: Fry spoonfuls of the batter until golden brown on both sides.
6: Serve with a drizzle of maple syrup and fresh fruit of your choice.

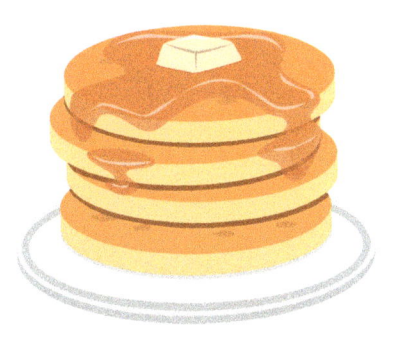

LIVING MINDFULLY

in SLEEP

Why do we need sleep?

Sleep is one of the most important aspects of our daily lives as the body is hard at work restoring, repairing and strengthening while we dream.

It is recommended that adults have between seven and nine hours of sleep each night. However, many people don't get enough sleep and this puts them at risk of increased anxiety levels, memory issues, diabetes, poor balance and high blood pressure, among other things.

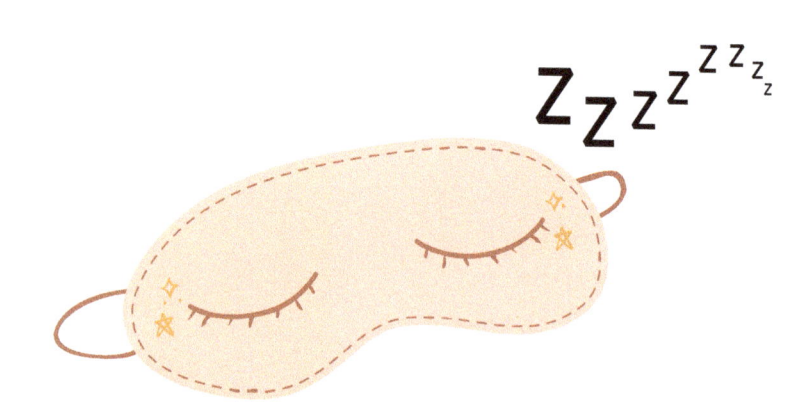

TIPS TO HELP YOU SLEEP Zzzz^{zz}

- Light a candle.
- Go to bed at the same time each night.
- Take a warm bath before bed.
- Write down a list of all the things you have to do the following day so that they aren't running through your mind when your head hits the pillow.
- Listen to gentle, soothing, relaxing music.
- Avoid watching TV or looking at your phone just before bedtime.
- Read for a short while before you turn off the lights.
- Have a warm, milky drink before going to bed.
- Use aromatherapy oils.
- Take at least 20 minutes of energetic exercise during the day.
- Keep the temperature in your bedroom cool.
- Draw the curtains and dim the lights.

Date _____ J F M A M J J A S O N D

this month's affirmation
I AM OPEN TO NEW WAYS OF IMPROVING MY HEALTH.

Intentions for the month

_____

_____

_____

Sleep

To do's

_____

_____

_____

_____

Thoughts & Feels

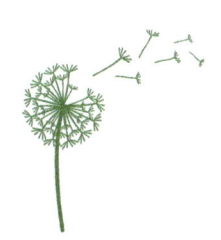

LIVING MINDFULLY

in STAR GAZING

Looking up at the sky on a clear night can help to shift your perspective. Often, problems that seem insurmountable don't feel quite so pressing when you gaze at the stars and realise just how vast the universe is.

Lying down and looking up at the night sky is also incredibly meditative as there is little to distract you visually when it's dark. If you look carefully, you'll be able to spot some of the constellations in our galaxy.

Stargazing is best done in a location where light pollution is minimal but sometimes, on a really clear night, you get a great view of the stars, even in an urban setting.

LIVING MINDFULLY
in STAR GAZING

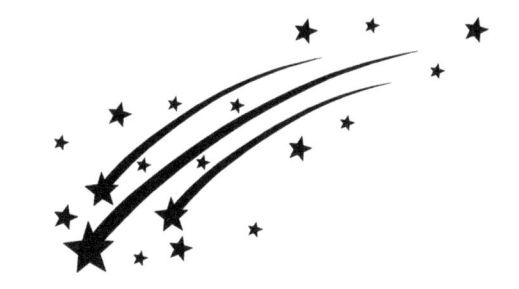

All you need is a sheet of plastic, (condensation can make the ground damp at night) and a comfortable mat, a cushion and warm clothes - the temperature drops at night, so make sure you have thick socks, a hat, gloves and a blanket, if required.

Immerse yourself in what you can see. Your eyes will adjust to the light, so stick with it and you'll be amazed by how much you can see.

Some of the things you might spot in the night sky:

Shooting Stars
Star Clusters - groups of stars
The Moon
Constellations - patterns of nearby stars

LIVING MINDFULLY

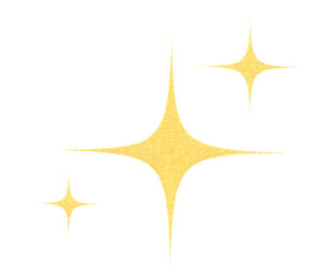

in STAR GAZING

Settle down, make yourself warm and comfortable and try this stargazing meditation:

- Choose a clear night and, if possible, find a place where there is minimal light pollution. If you live in a city, get as high up as you can. The best time to stargaze is during a crescent moon on a crisp winter's night.

- If you need a torch, use one with a red filter as it won't make it harder for your eyes to focus on the stars in the way that white or blue light will.

- Lie down on the ground, feel the weight of your body and notice how it makes contact with the earth. Appreciate the fact that the ground is supporting you - surrender to that feeling.

LIVING MINDFULLY

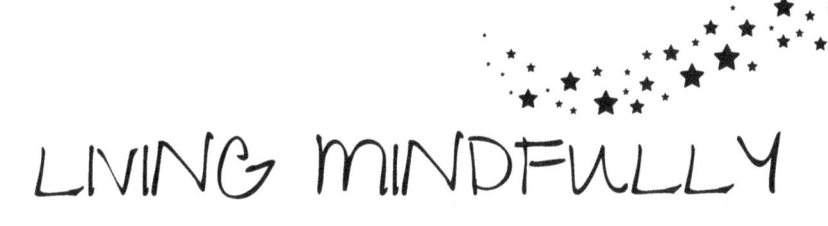

in STAR GAZING

- Take three deep breaths.

- Look at one patch of the sky.

- It takes 15 minutes for your eyes to adjust to the dark and the more you look, the more efficient they become.

- Appreciate the vastness of the galaxy beyond. Remind yourself that you are part of it.

- If you get sidetracked by other thoughts, bring your attention gently back to what you are looking at.

- You can close your eyes after a while, if this helps you reach a meditative state.

Date _____   J F M A M J J A S O N D

this month's affirmation
I AM AT PEACE WITH WHO I AM AS A PERSON.

Intentions for the month

_____

_____

_____

_____

To do's   Sleep

_____   _____

_____   _____

_____   _____

_____   _____

                              _____

                              _____

                              _____

Thoughts & Feels

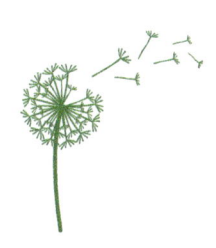

LIVING MINDFULLY

DECLUTTER & ORGANISE

Make more room for happiness

How do you feel when you're surrounded by a mess? Do you feel restless and unsettled? When disorder starts to creep in, do you feel a sense of 'outer control?'

Decluttering can help us feel more in control of our lives. It can create a feeling of sanctuary. A clear desk, tidy drawers, uncluttered shelves makes our spaces places of comfort and energy. We can revel in the pure pleasure of our possessions because we can see and reach everything easily.

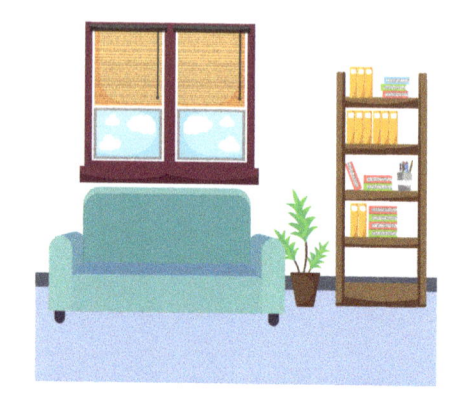

By improving the state of our surroundings, we can improve our state of mind.

LIVING MINDFULLY

MINDFUL CHORES

Everyday routine tasks, such as loading the dishwasher, cleaning, doing the laundry and tidying up can help challenge your assumptions and judgements about what is an ordeal - a tedious chore - and what is just a series of actions carried out in order to get something done.

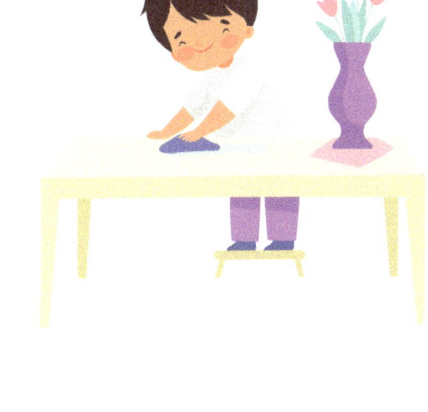

It is easy to make all sorts of negative judgements that are not necessary to do the job and get it done. None of these activities are good or bad. They are just activities. They are only annoying. tedious, boring or something to be resented if you think of them in that way. So, if such chores seem irritating to you, try doing them as an exercise in mindfulness. Instead of letting the time spent on these things be an unpleasant ordeal, engage yourself with those tasks without judgement.

Just do them without giving them any thought at all.

LIVING MINDFULLY
in TECHNOLOGY

Do A Tech Check

Technology can be great for helping you feel connected but if you're using it a lot then it can contribute to making you feel busy and stressed. Taking a break, even a short one, can help you relax.

Try turning your phone off for an hour (or a whole day if you're feeling brave.)

Step away from the TV or have an evening where you don't check emails or social networks. Use the time to relax doing something else.

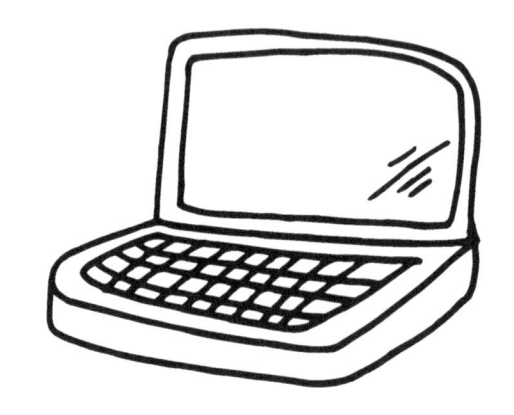

Identify times when you automatically turn to your phone, such as when travelling on a train and plan to do something else instead like listening to music, reading a book or doing a bit of colouring or drawing.

"If a cluttered desk is a sign of a cluttered mind, of what then is an empty desk a sign?"

- Albert Einstein

LIVING MINDFULLY

A LITTLE HOW-TO
Colour in the areas of your life that you've focused on lately.

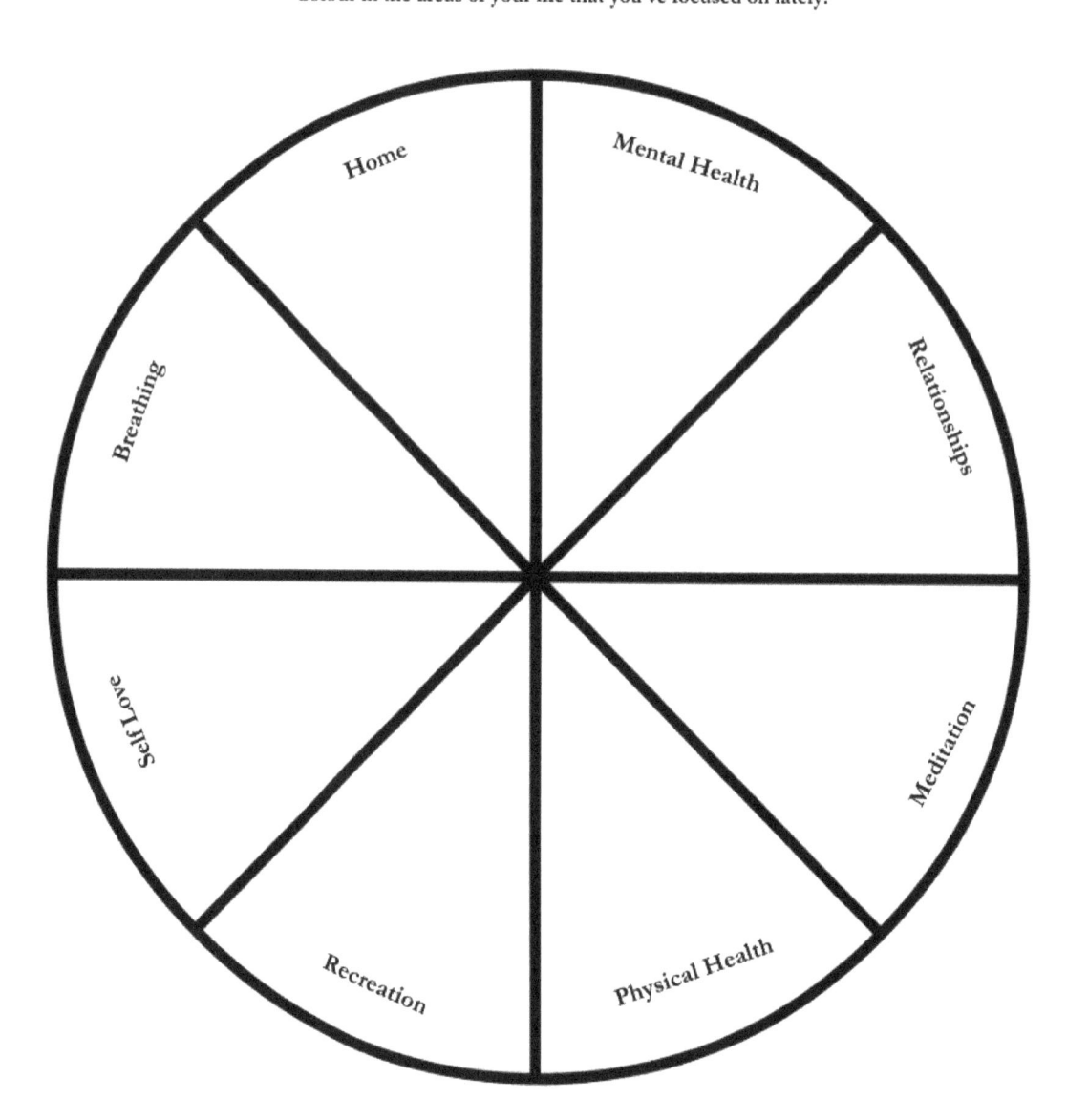

- Home
- Mental Health
- Relationships
- Meditation
- Physical Health
- Recreation
- Self Love
- Breathing

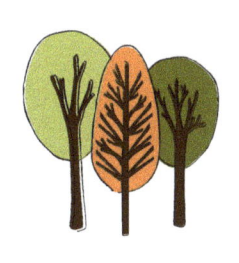

LIVING MINDFULLY
A MINDFUL REFLECTION

Take time to reflect and journal your own mindful moments, experiences and lessons learned.

LIVING MINDFULLY
in MINDFUL DRAWING

Take ten minutes to have a mindful experience with drawing.
Drawing inspired by music.

Drawing prompts:

1. Focus on your posture. Sit up straight and relax your shoulders.
2. Take a deep breath in for five seconds and then breathe out slowly for five seconds. Repeat this up to ten times.
3. Pick up a pen or pencil and take a moment to focus on your grip. If you find your grip is too tight, loosen it up. Experiment with different ways of holding your drawing tool.

Draw the music
- Play one of your favourite songs or types of music. Think about how different sounds might make a line do different things.
- Find a starting point on your paper and begin drawing. Let your line wander around the page and change direction or create shapes inspired by different sounds you hear.
- Try to keep drawing until the song ends.
- When you are done, think about how you might include colour.

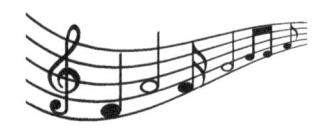

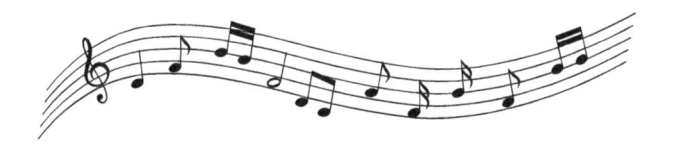

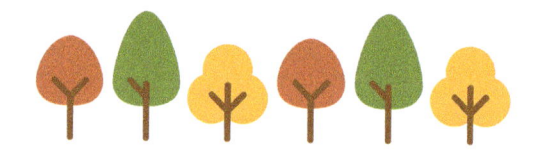

Bring Nature In

Bring back something from your next walk in nature
(whether that's the countryside, your garden or a park)
such as a leaf, fallen flower head, feather, toadstool,
pebble or piece of bark.

Take some time to really absorb its colours, patterns and
textures. Now take your pen and start drawing it on the page
opposite. Don't worry about trying to make it accurate.
It can be as abstract or wobbly as you like. The key here is to
allow all those things that you discovered about the object
to gently fill your mind and guide your hand as you draw.

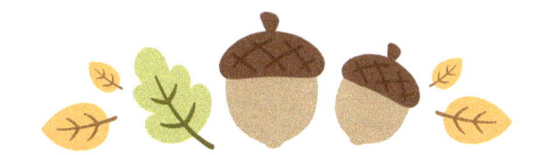

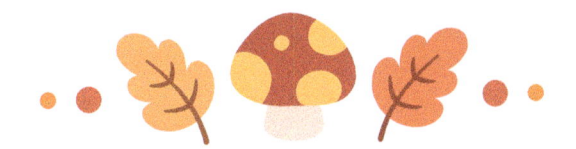

Date _____   J F M A M J J A S O N D

this month's affirmation
MY BODY IS A VESSEL OF WELLNESS.

Intentions for the month

_____

_____

_____

_____

                                      Sleep

To do's

                                  ☾ _____

_____   ☾ _____

_____   ☾ _____

                                  ☾ _____

_____   ☾ _____

_____   ☾ _____

                                  ☾ _____

Thoughts & Feels

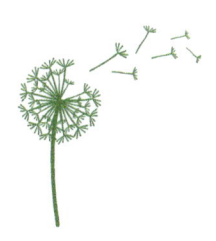

_____

_____

_____

_____

_____

_____

_____

LIVING MINDFULLY

continuing your journey

Mindfulness is an effective way to quieten the mind
and bring your attention to the present moment. This means letting go
of all the thoughts about the past or future.

Mindfulness is a state you enter when your mind is fully
engaged in whatever it is doing in the present moment.
Everybody is born with the ability to be mindful, however as
we grow older, the stresses and strains of everyday life
can take over and then we have to relearn how to access
this part of ourselves.

Remember, you can be mindful at any time of the day.
Live mindfully every day of your life and continue to
enjoy the journey of maintaining health and happiness.

"Walk as if you are kissing the Earth with your feet."

— Thich Nhat Hanh

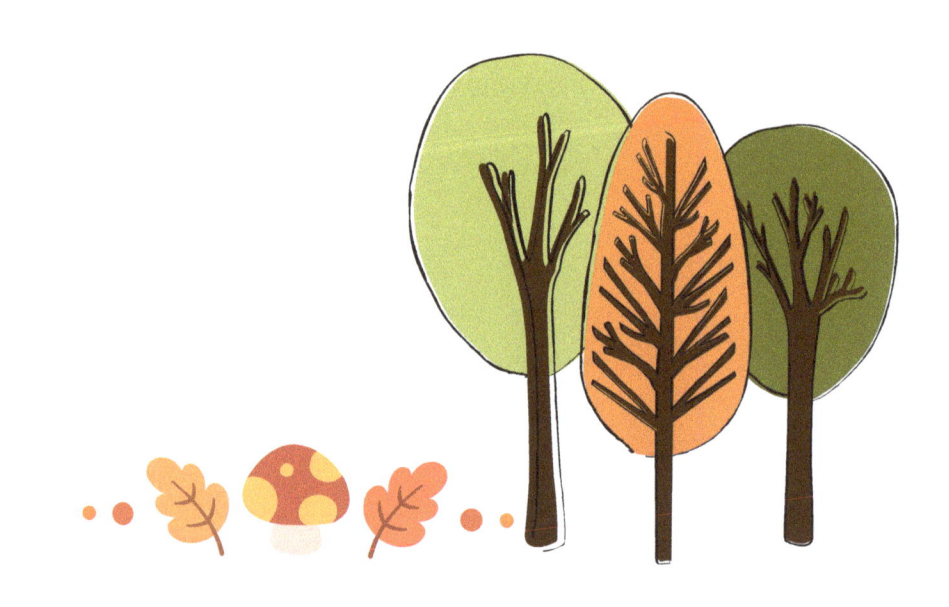

Milton Keynes UK
Ingram Content Group UK Ltd.
UKHW020049170224
437940UK00003B/8

9 781739 573041